ATKINS COOKBOOK

30 Quick And Easy Atkins Diet Recipes For Beginners,

Plan Your Low Carb Days With The New Atkins Diet Book,

Begin Weight Loss Revolution And Start Feeling Healthy Instantly

by Sandra Williams

TABLE OF CONTENTS

Introduction

I want to thank you and congratulate you for purchasing the book *Atkins Cookbook - 30 Quick And Easy Atkins Diet Recipes For Beginners*.

Atkins diet will help you to lose weight and reduce the risk of getting cardiovascular and metabolic diseases. It has been known to be effective in curing two types of diabetes. These are not just claims made by those who follow this diet. There have been countless research studies that have proven the efficacy of this type of diet. Research proves that the diet reduces risk factors, and can double the rate of weight loss, especially for those who have short term goals of losing weight.

The diet is particularly good for diabetics. The man who came up with the Atkins diet had type 2 diabetes and was overweight. He began his research, so that he could lose weight faster. He found that not only does this diet increase the rate of weight loss, but it can reverse the effects of type 2 diabetes.

Taking only the right amount of carbohydrates that the body needs, as well as increasing protein and fats is basically what this diet is about. Good fats are a better source of energy and they replace carbohydrates for that purpose.

Having less of carbohydrates in your diet reduces the risk of "Hyperinsulinism". Excess insulin will metabolize blood glucose and make you feel hungry. It is this hunger that leads to binge eating, especially on unhealthy food. Most traditional civilizations existing today indicate that humans have always survived on a diet full of protein. This means that humans evolved on this type of diet.

The best approach to this meal plan is to adopt it as a lifestyle. Be committed to it even when you reach your weight goals. Consistency and commitment are what you need to get to your fitness goals.

[Your Free Gift]

As a way of saying thanks for your purchase, I'm offering 2 free reports that are exclusive to my readers:

To check what are The 101 Tips That Burn Belly Fat Daily go to my page here:

=> http://projecteasylife.com/101tips <=

To see what are The 7 (Quick & Easy) Cooking Tricks To Banish Your Boring Diet go to my website here:

=> http://projecteasylife.com/7-tricks <=

DISCLAIMER: The purpose of this book is to provide information only. The information, though believed to be entirely accurate, is NOT a substitution for medical, psychological or professional advice, diagnosis or treatment. The author recommends that you seek the advice of your physician or other qualified health care provider to present them with questions you may have regarding any medical condition. Advice from your trusted, professional medical advisor should always supersede information presented in this book.

Chapter 1: An Atkins Diet Primer

Atkins Diet recipes are the answer to people looking to switch to low carb diet. Some people find that switching to a low carbohydrate, high protein diet, with no processed foods a little challenging. Therefore their current food sources are the exact opposite of what the Atkins diet demands.

Why exactly is it important to switch to a low carb diet plan? This meal plan can help you to lose weight much faster than people who are on a low fat diet. A study done on people on a low carbohydrate versus low fat meal plan showed that the rate of weight loss on an obese person, who was on a low carb meal plan, has doubled in comparison to a person who is on a low fat diet. The highest difference was seen after the first 3 months.

Low carb diet has other health benefits and is particularly known to prevent and reverse type 2 diabetes. According to the same study, it showed that people on this diet lost Non-HDL cholesterol more than those on the low fat meal plan.

A low carb diet can reduce your appetite significantly. One of the biggest problems people have today is binge eating. Processed foods, especially carbohydrates with high glycemic index, raise the blood glucoses quickly. Later, the level of blood glucoses goes down quickly and this leaves you hungry and weak.

Traditionally, many communities around the world had a diet similar to this meal plan. Studies have shown that the aboriginal communities of Canada have had more cases of cardiovascular diseases, after they adopted the modern high carbohydrate diet.

The Maasai in East Africa, who have maintained their culture, have a lower rate of high blood pressure, than other African communities who have adopted a high protein diet. Even though other Africans have a high incidence of high blood pressure at 20%, the Maasai prevalence has a much lower incidence of high blood pressure at 8.7%.

How Does It Work?

How does this meal plan help you to reduce weight loss? The main idea is to minimize the amount of sugars and starch that are on your plate. These foods are responsible for a higher production of insulin in your body.

Insulin is responsible for fat storage, plus water retention and sodium in the body. It is not uncommon for people, who switch to this diet plan, to lose a lot of weight in a short time. At this point the body begins to shed excess sodium and water.

How Much Carbs Should You Eat Per Day?

This is an important consideration for people, who want to adopt this meal plan. The simple answer is that it depends on the level of activity you engage in on a day to day basis. If you are very active, you will need more carbohydrates. People who live sedentary lifestyles should minimize their carbs intake. It is important to note that processed foods should be avoided as much as possible.

Phase 1

One way to start on this diet is to go about it in phases. In the first phase of the Atkins diet, you need to take a minimum of 18 grams of carbohydrates and 22 grams of carbohydrates. This is the amount necessary to provide the body with energy, while ensuring that it is primarily burning fat.

You have to continue doing this until you lose 15 pounds of fat. If followed to the letter, this can be achieved in the first two weeks. At this point you can move to Phase 2.

Phase 2

In Phase 2, the goal is to lose 10% of your total body weight. At this point, you need to reduce the amount of carbohydrates to about 25 grams. You also need to increase the amount of carbohydrates by 5 grams from this point on.

This phase is about avoiding losing track of the meal plan. So you need to adopt different kinds of foods and learn how to avoid unhealthy meals.

Phase 3

This phase involves strictly sticking to the meal plan. You may increase the carbohydrate intake from between 5 and 10 grams. This phase is important, if you want to reach your weight loss goal. You should take this phase seriously.

Phase 4

The last phase should be followed until your weight loss goal is achieved. At this point, it is important to note that this meal plan is not a diet plan. You must continue with what you started. This phase involves adopting the meal plan as a lifestyle.

It is important to note that the carbohydrate intake recommended above is ideal for overweight people who are leading a sedentary life. However, people who are leaner and active need about 100 to 150 grams of carbohydrates. On the other hand, people who are not overweight and not very active, and need to get to lose weight, may take between 50 and 75 grams of carbohydrates per day.

Protein Intake

Since you will be taking smaller amounts of carbohydrates, you need to increase your protein consumption. Protein helps to boost your metabolism. It also has another advantage in that it kills your appetite significantly. These two benefits can help you lose weight quickly.

But what proteins do you need? It all depends if you are a vegetarian or not. Vegetarians may need to be more careful of the types of protein in their diet.

Myths

There are certain myths about this meal plan, which often come from misunderstanding of nutrition, as well as the parts of the Atkins diet. Here are some of them.

All Carbohydrates Are Bad And Fattening

The main aim of the Atkins diet is to reduce the amount of carbohydrate you take per meal or per day. The aim of this meal plan is to limit the intake of carbohydrates, in order to lose weight. However, it is important to realize that not all carbohydrates are bad. You also need to note that this meal plan does not entirely prohibit the intake of carbohydrates.

Not all carbohydrates are fattening. But there are some that must be avoided at all costs. Ideally, processed foods should be eliminated completely from your diet. Most of the processed carbohydrates have a high glycemic index.

What foods with high glycemic index do is to raise the blood sugar level, and then your blood sugar nose dives. This leaves you hungry and feeling weak. These foods also make you more prone to binge eating and encourage an obsessive craving for food.

The Meal Plan Must Be Ketogenic

In low carb meal plan, the term ketogenic is used to refer to very low levels of carbohydrates that are usually the aim of this plan. A ketogenic diet requires that you take below 50 grams of carbohydrates per day.

However, this meal plan does not necessarily have to be ketogenic. It can be higher than this, and the carbohydrate intake can be as high as 150 grams per day. It all depends on how active you are. If you feel you cannot handle low levels of carbohydrates, you may opt to take more carbs and exercise more to ensure that more carbohydrates are burned.

Low Carb Diet Automatically Leads To Weight Loss

It may happen that some people do not watch what they eat outside of this meal plan. That means that they binge eat in between meals. You need to watch what you eat and avoid snacks, which add to the total amount of carbohydrate intake.

Most of these snacks may be processed carbs, which reverse the gains made by this meal plan. Nuts and other 'healthy' snacks should be avoided, unless they are part of the meal plan and do not contribute to binge eating. If you fail to observe this rule, you will not only fail to lose weight, but gain more weight in the process.

Eggs Are Unhealthy

Eggs are among the single most nutritious foods you can find. Eggs have almost all the nutrients needed by humans. They are also relatively cheap, so they are among the top choice for people looking to adopt the Atkins diet.

The problem with eggs is that the yolk has high levels of cholesterol. Most people avoid eggs for this reason. However, this fear is as a result of a misconception on cholesterol intake. To understand why eggs are not risky, it is important to look at how the body controls and maintains the required levels of cholesterol. Your body needs considerable amount of cholesterol every day. The cell membrane makes use of cholesterol to create a barrier. It is also an important component for hormones like testosterone and estrogen. Your body requires 200 to 300 milligrams of cholesterol every day.

What if the body is not getting the required amounts of cholesterol? When this happens, the liver produces the required amounts of cholesterol. According to scientists, whether you take in the required amounts or not, the levels remain the same in the body. The only difference is in the type of cholesterol produced.

Quick Tips to Make the Most of Atkins Diet

Carbohydrates

Avoid processed carbohydrates. Take complex carbs. However, if you are going to work out in the morning, ensure you take enough carbs and water before you work out. The body takes longer to convert complex carbs to energy, so you will have to take it at least an hour before the work out. Failing to hydrate and give the body energy is one of the reasons why people end up feeling lethargic for the rest of the day.

Drinks

Green tea: Green tea is one of the healthiest drinks you can adopt in place of black tea, or coffee. It has very powerful antioxidants, which are very effective for reducing the chances of getting cancer.

Wine: You can take a glass or two of wine with your food. However, you need to ensure that you eliminate beer and other drinks with a lot of calories from your diet.

Milk and dairy: Limit milk and other dairy products. This can raise insulin levels and increase the amount of fat that your body chooses to store. This is counterproductive, since it is the exact opposite of what you are trying to achieve.

Water: There is no consensus about how much water you should drink per day. However, most experts agree that 1.5 to 2 liters of water per day is enough. Taking small amounts of water throughout the day is more effective than taking large amounts at once. Water keeps your skin smooth, body healthy, and there is also evidence from studies that it greatly influences your mood.

Ordering at the Restaurant

You can make quick orders at your favorite restaurant without having to over analyze everything you order.

Vegetables: Opt for more vegetables than potatoes and starchy foods.

Proteins: Make sure that you have either fish or meat in your plate.

Exercise

Consider taking advantage of the high protein intake to increase muscle mass and increase your metabolic rate.

Weight training: This increases muscle mass and ensures that the body is utilizing the protein that you take. The more weight training you do per week, the more proteins you can take. It is advisable to structure your exercise regimen such that you eat proteins before you work out and carbs after that.

Resistance training: This increases your metabolism, muscle mass, and also facilitates protein synthesis, which ensures that you are not left with excess proteins in the body. Eat complex carbs at least an hour before training to ensure that you get the energy needed during the workout.

Exercise and rest: Rest is an important part of the exercise that is sometimes ignored by those who are too keen to get results. You should work out for 4 days of the week consecutively, and then rest for 4 days. This is an ideal system favored by athletes and body builders.

Know the Ingredients

It is important to understand the ingredients of the things that you buy, as well as what the label says. For instance, eggs can be omega 3 enriched and beef can be from grass fed cows. It is imperative to understand the implications of this as they affect quality, nutrition, and even taste.

Chapter 2: Egg Recipes

Eggs have all the nutrients you need and they are amongst the cheapest ingredients for Atkins diet. They are also very good sources of protein. Here are some recipes that will make taking eggs interesting.

Crustless Quiche Lori-iane

Ingredients:

- Chopped tomatoes about a quarter of a cup
- An equal amount of chopped tomatoes
- A tablespoon of Oregano
- 2 ounce of canned green chilies drained and chopped
- A small piece of garlic minced
- Shredded cheddar cheese ½ cup
- Tablespoon paprika

Instructions:

1. Preheat the oven to about 300^0 Fahrenheit. You'll need to find a glass pan or pie plate and oil it.
2. Break the eggs into a bowl. Whisk the eggs and add any cream of your choice. Add the other ingredients such as: tomatoes, onions cheese, Oregano, and Paprika.
3. Add the mixture onto the glass plate and place it in an oven using a baking sheet.
4. Bake the mixture.

Egg Muffins

You can make 6 egg muffins with this recipe. Note that the most important part of the recipe is the eggs and the green onions. You can experiment with other ingredients. The muffins can also be refrigerated for about a week.

Ingredients:

- 6 Eggs in muffin pans, either silicon, or metallic muffin pans

- 1 or 2 tablespoon salt (or any other seasoning that you feel is good with eggs)

- 1-2 containers ground low fat cheese

- 3 green onions diced into small pieces

- You may also use vegetables to reduce fat content, some of the vegetables you can use are zucchini mushrooms, and broccoli

Instructions:

1. Preheat the stove to 370^0 Fahrenheit.

2. Use the silicon muffin pans or tins, and place the eggs in each of the cups. Ensure that the muffins do not get stuck by using a nonstick spray (you may opt to use coconut or olive oil instead). Most regular muffin pans may require paper liners.

3. On the base of each of the cups, cover the bottom of the cup with the ingredients you are using except eggs. Add green onions, cheese, meat, and any chopped vegetables that you may opt to use.

4. Fill each cup and leave the upper 1/3 for the eggs. Break the eggs and pour over the mixture until the cup is almost full.

5. Add any seasoning of your choice and cream.

6. Blend the mixture slowly with a folk. Place in the oven for about 30 minutes. When done, the muffins will rise and be slightly brown.

Steamed Cinnamon Coconut Milk Egg Custard

Ingredients:

- 2 eggs
- 2 egg yolks (at room temperature)
- 1/3 glass granulated sweetener
- 2 glasses unsweetened coconut milk
- 1/4 tablespoon salt
- 1/4 tablespoon ground cinnamon
- 6 pieces (7oz) ramekins

Instructions:

1. Fill a heating tray with water and preheat in the oven to 300° Fahrenheit.
2. Gently whisk eggs and egg yolks in a huge vessel, and then blend in some sweetener.
3. Add cinnamon and salt to the coconut drain and blend well.
4. Add coconut milk to the egg mixture and blend well, then sifter the custard mixture into a measuring mug or a container.
5. Put the mixture into arranged ramekins and leave only 1/3 of the cup empty, after that cover with aluminum foil.
6. Cook in the preheated broiler for about 30 minutes.
7. Switch off the oven and let it stay in the oven for an additional 10 minutes.
8. Serve warm or chilled.

Eggs and Veggies Fried in Coconut Oil

This is a simple breakfast you can prepare. It is ideal for people, who do not have a lot of time in the morning to prepare an elaborate meal.

Ingredients:

- 3 or 4 medium sized eggs

- Coconut oil

- One tablespoon pepper

- 1 tablespoon salt

- Frozen vegetable mix of choice (e.g. Spinach, cauliflower and green beans)

Instructions:

1. Add an adequate amount of coconut oil onto the frying pan and let it heat up.

2. Add the vegetable mix; let it remain in the pan for about a minute.

3. After the vegetables have thawed, add the eggs.

4. Add the eggs letting them mix with the salt, black pepper, and any other spices.

5. Continue stirring the mixture until the eggs are cooked. Ensure that the egg is not overcooked.

Bacon and Eggs

This is another breakfast meal that is easy to prepare. It is high in protein. It may not be the best breakfast for people trying to avoid processed foods, but it qualifies as a suitable high protein diet.

Ingredients:

- Bacon

- 3 or so eggs

- Salt and any seasoning you prefer

Instructions:

1. Begin by frying the bacon slowly in the pan. Turn down the heat, so that it fries slowly without getting burned.

2. Add the eggs. The eggs should fry in the oil produced by the bacon. If the amount of oil in the pan is not enough, you may add coconut oil.

3. Add seasoning and spices while frying (this is optional and depends on your taste).

4. Add tomatoes or vegetables as a salad.

Cheese Omelet with Broccoli

This is an easy breakfast meal that you can make in a minute or two. Perfect high protein breakfast for when you are in a hurry. Serving for 2 people.

Ingredients:

- 2 eggs
- 2 cups of broccoli
- ½ cup of egg whites
- 1 tablespoon olive oil
- Salt and fresh pepper
- A small amount of grated cheese
- 1 tablespoon pepper

Instructions:

1. Use a container to mix all the ingredients.
2. Mix the ingredients together.
3. Add the eggs, egg whites, cheese salt, and pepper together.
4. Use greased tins or muffin plates and pour the ingredients into four or so cups.
5. Put the tins into a preheated oven (to about 375^0 Fahrenheit). After 20 minutes your egg broccolis omelet should be cooked.
6. You can place the remaining omelets in a fridge and simply microwave them when you need them.

Asian Omelet

Ingredients:

- 2 eggs

- 1 teaspoon of soy sauce

- 1 teaspoon pepper

- 1 teaspoon butter

- Salt to taste

- Spicy Cabbages or vegetables such as kales

Instructions:

1. Heat the butter in a non-stick pan.

2. Mix the soy sauce and eggs together. Add only a small amount of salt, since the soy sauce is normally salty.

3. Add the mixture to the pan.

4. Heat the vegetables in a microwave and add it on top of the mixture on the pan.

5. Turn the egg and ensure it is evenly cooked.

6. It is now ready to serve.

Sausage and Eggs

This is another easy meal you can make for breakfast. The vegetables have powerful anti-oxidants and the sausage and eggs will give you the proteins you need.

Ingredients:

- Find dark green vegetables such as spinach or kale

- 4 or 5 eggs

- Raw sausages cut into pieces

- Spice it up with parsley, rosemary, or any other herb

Instructions:

1. Start by cutting the vegetables into long strips.

2. Sauté the vegetables in a pan for a few minutes.

3. Place the sausages in the pan and stir the mixture.

4. Add the eggs and the herbs.

5. Pour the mixture into a baking pan. Place the mixture into an oven preheated at 375^0 Fahrenheit. Bake for about 20 minutes.

Cheese Omelet

You can make omelets, by either whisking the egg (simple omelet) or whisking the egg and the yolk separately (fluffy omelet). This depends on your taste.

Ingredients:

- 4 eggs

- Chopped parsley, a teaspoon or less

- 5 teaspoons of grated cheddar cheese

Instructions:

1. Decide whether you want simple or fluffy omelet and prepare them as stated above.

2. Add the egg into the pan and fry for minute.

3. Add cheddar cheese and parsley.

Chapter 3: Atkins Diet Phase One Recipes

Phase one is the induction phase of the Atkins meal plan. In this phase, you need to limit the amount of carbohydrates especially, if you are doing it for weight loss. Here are some of the recipes you can use to start you off in phase one.

Grilled Chicken

Serving for 3.

Ingredients:

- 3 chicken breasts, boneless and skinless
- ¼ cup plain yoghurt
- 1 garlic clove crushed
- 2 tablespoons of ground ginger
- 1 tablespoon lemon juice
- 1 cucumber seeded and peeled

Instructions:

1. Place chicken bosoms in a zip container to marinate it. Mix for a minute or two by massaging the chicken.

2. Place this mixture in the refrigerator for about 4-5 hours. Take the breasts out of the marinade, grill them until it turns clear. It should be ready in about 20 minutes.

3. At this point you may use the Tzatziki sauce on the chicken. The mixture should be refrigerated for a few hours.

4. Cut the chicken across then use the Tzatziki sauce before serving.

Simple Chicken Soup

This recipe is for about 12 generous servings.

Ingredients:

- 1 full chicken should ideally be 4 or 5 lbs.

- 4 liters of water

- 3 big celery stalks

- 3 fairly big carrots

- 3 sizeable garlic cloves

- 1 big onion or 2-3 of small ones

- 3 dried sound clears out

- 6 stems of thyme

- ¼ cup of chopped parsley

- 1 tablespoon salt or other seasoning of your choice

- 2 teaspoons black pepper to taste

- You may add small amounts of grain particularly complex carbohydrates, such as 1 cup of barley or brown rice

Instructions:

1. Begin by cleaning the chicken. Wash it thoroughly ensuring that you remove all the organs inside. You may use some of the organs as part of the soup, if you wish. Some people may choose to remove the skin and chicken fat. Uproot and discard the chicken fat that is regularly stopped inside the lower hole of the chicken around the

thighs, you do not have to remove this fat; it can be a good source of energy, if you are not going to add grains in the soup. Otherwise you can wrap it and use it later for frying. Fill up the pot with water and put in chicken.

2. Add salt and pepper; wrap thyme and bay leaves in some knotted cheesecloth for easier removal later, then add to the pot. Wash carrots, remove the unwanted parts, cut one in the middle, and the other two into unequal parts. Wash celery, remove the unwanted parts, and cut one in the middle and the other two into unequal parts. Ensure you remove the green part from the celery. You may now peel the onion, remove the unwanted parts of the onion, leave it as it is and do not cut it into pieces. Peel the garlic cloves; do not cut it into pieces. Now place everything in a pot with water and the chicken. Cover the pot. Let it simmer for some time as you stir it from time to time. Keep stirring to prevent some of the ingredients from getting stuck at the bottom.

3. You will need to stir the mixture slowly in the pot from time to time. The chicken should cook for 1 hour 30 minutes to 2 hours. When fully cooked, the chicken will turn white. Remove the leaves from the thyme. Carefully put the chicken pieces with folks or spoons, put in a bowl, and let it remain away from the stove for about 20 minutes.

4. Separate the pieces of meat using folks, knives, or two spoons. Break the bones to enrich the broth.

5. Let the chicken cool, take out the parts of the cooked carrot and celery and cut them into pieces. Add some parsley. Blend the mixture. Get out your nourishment processor; scoop out vegetables with a big spoon. However, the carrot and celery you simply cut. A portion of the onion may have broken into smaller pieces, so incorporate those bigger pieces, likewise seek for the garlic, which may have broken down, so don't stress if you can't seem to find it. Add veggies to your processor. Pulse the mixture first for about 10 seconds to get it going, then puree until veggies start to

melt and descend within the highest point of the processor for 20 seconds.

6. Include the vegetables and place them in a soup pot. Add whole grained carbs such as brown rice, wheat, or you may also opt to go for pasta. Mix well. At the point when the chicken is cool and simpler to handle, take a couple of expansive dim meat pieces and/or about ½ of a chicken breast, put in the processor, and pulse for 15 seconds. Add sliced chicken again to the soup. Take the rest of the chicken apart with your fingers, ensuring that you peel off from the bones, and tear it into relatively small pieces of meat. Add the chicken again to the soup. Warm for a few minutes and blend completely.

NB: You can remove excess fat from this soup by simply letting it cool. When cool, you may whiff off the excess fat flowing at the top of the soup.

Chapter 4: Fish Recipes

Fish is one of the best proteins that you can choose to have as part of your Atkins diet. It has important nutrients, which you do not often find in other dishes that you eat on a day to day basis. It has vitamin D and Riboflavin (B2). It is also rich in calcium, magnesium, iron, and phosphorus.

Omega 3 fatty acids found in fish are good fats. They facilitate brain development and help improve heart health. They also reduce the risk of heart disease, Alzheimer, ADHD, Dementia, and diabetes.

Catfish in Creamy Shallot Sauce

Catfish is relatively easier to cook compared to other types of fish. This meal will leave your taste buds with the buttery taste of delicious catfish prepared in shallot sauce.

Ingredients:

- 1 fillet of catfish
- 1 tablespoon olive oil (or coconut oil)
- 2 tablespoons butter
- 1 shallot sliced into small pieces
- Approximately 4 tablespoons of lemon juice
- ¼ cup of coconut milk

Instructions:

1. Lift the fillet and pat it and let it dry.

2. Sauté the sliced shallot for half a minute.

3. Add 2 tablespoons of butter.

4. Let the butter melt then add the fillet.

5. Let it fry on either side for a few minutes then turn it over.

6. Remove the fillets from the pan and add lemon juice over it.

7. Add coconut onto the pan and let it heat up for a minute or two before putting back the fillet and then stir.

8. In about 3 minutes the catfish fillet will be ready to serve.

Grilled Fish in Grape Tomato Sauce

This is a great Atkins fish recipe for those who love tomato sauce. Depending on the amount of carbohydrates you are limiting yourself to, you can eat it with brown rice or pasta. Without the extra carbohydrates, this meal has less than 10 grams of carbohydrates.

Ingredients:

- 6 ground cloves of garlic

- 1 tablespoon of olive oil

- 1 fresh pepper

- Salt to taste

- 4 pieces of tilapia

- Fresh basil chopped

Instructions:

1. Use a large pan and add olive oil. Let it heat before adding garlic.

2. Let the garlic fry on the pan, until it is golden brown.

3. Once it turns to golden brown, reduce the heat and add tomatoes, and pepper.

4. Let this sauce simmer a little then add salt. Wait for about 15 minutes then add basil.

5. After another 5 minutes add fish. Let it simmer for a while. You may grill the fish for a few minutes, until it turns golden brown.

Baked Tilapia

Serving for one person.

Ingredients:

- About 7 ounces of tilapia
- 1 teaspoon of chili pepper
- 1 teaspoon oregano
- 2 teaspoons of lemon juice
- A pinch of cayenne pepper

Instructions:

1. Mix chili pepper, cayenne, oregano, and salt in one small container.

2. Melt butter and transfer it into a shallow pan. Add lemon onto the butter.

3. Poor the spice mixture into the butter and lemon mixture.

4. Add the fillet into the bowl containing the mixture. Massage the fillets into the spice, and lemon butter mixture. Ensure the mixture is spread evenly on all the fillets.

5. Transfer it into a casserole.

6. Preheat the oven to 450^0 Fahrenheit. In about 15 minutes the fillets should be flaky and soft. They are now ready to serve.

Crispy Baked Fish

Ingredients:

- 16 ounce fish fillets
- ¼ cup milk
- 2 teaspoon vinegar
- 1 tale spoon honey mustard
- 1 teaspoon salt
- 1 small chopped garlic
- 1 teaspoon pepper
- ½ teaspoon thyme
- 1 teaspoon cayenne pepper
- 1 teaspoon paprika

Instructions:

1. Take the ¼ cup of milk and add vinegar and honey mustard. Mix it thoroughly and let it rest for 15 minutes.

2. Mix cornmeal chopped onions, paprika, cayenne, and all the spices listed.

3. In a sizeable bowl, add milk, and then fillets. After a few seconds remove and place the fillets into the cornmeal and spices mixture that you had added later.

4. Apply some olive oil on the pan you will be using to avoid the mixture sticking when baking.

5. Place the pan on moderate heat and let it cook for about 5 minutes as you turn. The fish will be ready, once it is flaky and soft. You may serve after squeezing lemon.

Crusted Salmon with Herbs

Ingredients:

- 6oz of salmon fillets

- 2 tablespoons of dried parsley

- 1 full tablespoon coconut floor

- 1 tablespoon pepper

- 1 tablespoon salt

- 1 tablespoon olive oil

- Some dijon mustard cream

Instructions:

1. Place the fillet on a foil.

2. Preheat the oven to 450^0 Fahrenheit.

3. Add olive oil onto the fillet then add the mustard and massage.

4. Create a mixture of dried parsley, salt and pepper.

5. Now add the mixture onto the salmon and pat.

6. Place the salmon into the oven for about 12 to 15 minutes.

7. Make a vegetable salad and top the crusted salmon, when it is fully baked.

Sautéed Salmon

Ingredients:

- 4 salmon fillets of about 6 ounces
- 4 tablespoon of butter not mixed up
- A teaspoon of lemon juice
- 1 tablespoon of pepper
- Salt to taste
- Some cream

Instructions:

1. Use a pan to melt 3 tablespoons of butter.
2. Place the salmon on the pan and sauté for 10 minutes turning to ensure it is cooked evenly.
3. Add salt and pepper to taste.
4. Use a spoon to sprinkle some lemon juice on the salmon.
5. After a minute or so, remove and place on a plate.
6. Add few spoonfuls of butter and cream.
7. Place the salmon back onto the pan, and let it cook for about 2 minutes.
8. Once cooked, you may serve the salmon with several slices of lemon.

Spiced Tilapia

Ingredients:

- 8 ounces of Tilapia fillets
- 3 spoonfuls of olive oil
- 3 garlic cloves cut into small pieces
- Salt to taste
- 1 teaspoon of pepper
- 1 squeezed lemon
- Chopped parsley

Instructions:

1. Mix the salt and pepper together.
2. Apply the mixture onto the fillets.
3. Place oil in a pan and heat moderately.
4. Let the pan heat before placing the fillets.
5. Turn the fillets from time to time, until they begin to change color.
6. Add some garlic to the fillets.
7. Continue frying the fish in the pan. When cooked it should peel easily, when you poke the fillet with a knife or a folk.
8. Also, for better tasting garlic tilapia, let the fillets continue frying slowly until the garlic is golden brown. However, you should ensure that the garlic doesn't turn black, i.e. get burned.
9. You may now squeeze some lemon juice over the fillets and serve.

Chapter 5: Beef Based Recipes

A lot has been said about beef in the past, especially in relation to dieting. For a long time beef was thought to be very unhealthy. It turns out to be one of the best sources of certain nutrients that people around the world are deficient of.

60% of humans do not take adequate quantities of iron in the body. Beef is one of the best sources. Selenium, vitamin b112, and zinc are also found in beef.

When choosing beef for Atkins diet, ensure that it is lean. Avoid very fatty beef, since it is not the best source of fat. Ensure you get the right amount of protein, but do not over eat beef. Most adults need slightly less than 60 grams of protein in their diet daily.

Eat smaller portions of meat over time, then one big portion of meat in one sitting. Some of the recipes mentioned here are great for people going through the first phase.

Pineapple Meatballs

A delicious meatball beef meal, with added pineapple flavor.

Ingredients:

- 1 medium sized green pepper cut into sizeable piece
- 5 tablespoons of white vinegar
- 5 tablespoons pineapple flavor
- ½ cup of granular Splenda
- 14 ounce beef broth
- 2 tablespoons soy sauce

- 1 carrot sliced horizontally

- 1 or 1½ teaspoon of xanthan gum

- Salt to taste

Instructions:

1. Add the meatballs, sliced carrots, and green pepper together in a pot.

2. Add and mix the spices and the remaining ingredients except the xanthan gum.

3. As you mix the ingredients add small amounts of the xanthan gum and mix. Keep repeating this until the result is a thick meatball. Do not add too much of the gum at once. Also do not exceed the amount, so keep checking to ensure you get it right.

Spinach Beef Cake

This is a recipe that has adequate amounts of vegetables and beef. It is ideal for Atkins phase one (induction phase).

Ingredients:

- 2 lbs. of minced meat
- 2 medium sized onions
- 2 eggs
- 3/4 lbs. spinach thawed and drained
- 4 ounce canned mushrooms
- 4 ounces mozzarella cheese
- 1 ounce parmesan cheese
- 2 tablespoon melted butter
- 1 teaspoon pepper
- Salt to taste
- 1 tablespoon garlic

Instructions:

1. Heat the pan and add a little bit of coconut or olive oil.
2. Add the onions and let them be brown.
3. Add beef to the onions and wait it for a few minutes till it changes color.
4. Mix the rest of the ingredients, and then add butter.
5. Place the mixture in a casserole, and then bake it in an oven at 375^0 for 30 minutes.

Fried Chicken Breasts with Butter

You can add other ingredients other than butter depending on your taste.

Ingredients:

- 3 tablespoons of Butter
- A substantial amount of Chicken breasts
- 2-3 teaspoons of garlic powder
- Green vegetables as salad
- Curry powder
- Black Pepper
- Salt to taste

Instructions:

1. Ensure that the chicken breasts are cut into small pieces.
2. Place the pan on the stove, add butter, and turn up the heat.
3. As the butter melts, add chicken breasts.
4. Mix the salt, garlic powder, and pepper.
5. Add the mix onto the chicken breasts and turn them as the fry.
6. Add the cut vegetables onto the cooked vegetables and serve.

Minced Meat with Bell Peppers

Ingredients:

- Coconut oil

- Onions sliced into small pieces

- Minced beef

- Salt to taste

- 1 tablespoon pepper

- Chili powder

- Vegetables such as spinach and kales cut into sizeable pieces

Instructions:

1. Heat up the pan and add some coconut oil to it.

2. Let it heat up and add the onions.

3. Let the onions turn into a golden brown color then add the minced beef.

4. Add the pepper and chili powder.

5. Add the cut vegetables and turn the minced beef and vegetables, then add bell pepper.

6. In about 10 minutes the food should be cooked.

Baked Meatballs

Ingredients:

- Low cup ketchup about 1/8 of a cup

- Minced meat 16 ounces

- 1 teaspoon dried onion flakes

- A pinch of pepper

- 1 egg

- 2 ounce shredded cheese

- Salt to taste

- Glaze

Instructions:

1. Preheat oven to 450^0 Fahrenheit.

2. Place foil on a loaf pan. Line up the minced meat mixed with all the ingredients on the foil, minus the glaze.

3. Cover with the foil, and then apply the glaze over the minced meat.

4. Place the mixture in an oven.

5. After about 15 minutes at 450^0. Then reduce the temperature to 350^0 for the next 50 minutes.

Spiced Minced Beef

Ingredients:

- 4 teaspoons of unsalted butter
- 1 onion sliced and peeled
- 1 teaspoon of turmeric
- 1 teaspoon of chili
- 2 cloves of garlic cut into small pieces
- ½ teaspoon cumin
- 1 teaspoon of ground coriander
- 16 ounces of minced beef

Instructions:

1. Heat a large pan and add the butter, letting it melt.
2. Add the small pieces of onions onto the pan and let it turn golden brown slowly.
3. When it turns golden brown add the turmeric, chili, and cumin.
4. Reduce the heat and turn everything slowly for 2-3 minutes on the pan.
5. Add the minced beef onto the pan; let it cook as you stir from time to time.
6. Once the beef is cooked, you can drain the excess grease and serve.

Spicy Minced Beef

This meal is great for the first phase of Atkins meal plan.

Ingredients:

- 1 pound of minced beef
- 1 onion cut into small pieces
- Cut 1 green pepper, and 1 red pepper into strips
- A teaspoon of grated ginger
- 3 teaspoons of butter

Instructions:

1. Using a large pan, add some butter, and then heat up the pan.
2. Add the onions and let the onions turn golden brown.
3. Add the meat, and then sprinkle the red and green pepper as you turn the meat.
4. If there is excess grease on the pan, pour it out.
5. Continue cooking the meat, until it is crispy and brown.
6. It works best with soy sauce and red pepper, but you may add any other sauce and salads according to your tastes.

Minced Meat Filling

Ingredients:

- 1 Teaspoon thyme
- A dash of rosemary
- 2 small cups of sliced tomatoes
- 2 cups cabbages chopped
- A generous amount of tomato sauce
- 2 cans beef bouillon
- 2 cups green beans
- ½ teaspoon of pepper
- Salt

Instructions:

1. Heat the pan and then add the olive oil. Let it heat then add chopped onions.
2. Place the meat on the olive oil and let it brown for some time.
3. Add the rest of the ingredients.
4. Continue stirring the mixture in low or medium heat until the meat is cooked.

Burgundy Beef Stew

For this recipe, it is advisable to use low carb baking mix.

Ingredients:

- ¼ cup of baking powder
- 4-5 chopped onions
- 3 lbs. beef cut into cubes
- Reasonable amounts of chopped carrots
- 3 tablespoons of olive oil
- Chopped celery
- 2 garlic cloves
- 2 cups red wine
- 1 tablespoon fresh thyme
- Fresh parsley chopped
- ¼ lbs. bacon slices

Instructions:

1. Coat the beef with salt and pepper first. Then add the baking powder.
2. Cook bacon in a pan, until it is crisp, and then remove the bacon.
3. Using the same pan, use the bacon fat that remains. Add brown beef cubes. Add onions carrots and celery. Add garlic.
4. Add wine and let it boil. Add beef, then the beef broth. Reduce heat and add thyme and parsley. After 30 minutes, the beef should be cooked.
5. Remove beef and serve with bacon.

Chapter 6: Vegetarian Recipes

Plant based proteins are considered to be more heart friendly, than fats got from animal proteins such as beef. Even though plant proteins lead to the same amount of weight loss, it reduces risk factors that cause heart disease. The only problem with plant based protein is that it does not always have all the proteins you need.

If you are a vegetarian, or you simply want to get more of your protein from plants, you need to ensure that the macro nutrients balance of the plant based protein is done right. You need to ensure you are getting all the proteins your body needs.

Peanut Butter Balls

These are protein balls made from a lot of peanut butter and whey. Whey is a great source of protein.

Ingredients:

- 1 cup peanut butter (preferably peanut butter that is sugar and additives free)

- 1 teaspoon vanilla

- Slightly over 1 cup of whey protein powder

- You may add some artificial sweetener to taste (preferably one without a lot of additives)

- Crushed nuts (optional)

Instructions:

1. Place the ingredients in a medium sized bowl and mix.

2. You can use a mixer or a spoon to mix all the ingredients together except the crushed nuts.

3. After you have thoroughly mixed the ingredients, roll them into balls.

4. You may place the crushed nuts and roll the balls, if you opt to add crushed nuts.

5. You can add little bit of artificial sweetener. Make sure that you do not add excessive amounts of it to avoid stickiness.

Easy Pimento Cheese

This is not a strictly vegan recipe. It is however, suitable for those looking for low carb recipes with no meat. It is very easy to prepare and does not involve any boiling, frying or baking.

Ingredients:

- 1 cup of shredded cheese

- 2 ounces of pimento pepper cut into small pieces (some people prefer smaller pieces of pimento, so you may run it through a chopper)

- About 8 ounces of salad dressing

- 1 teaspoon of pepper

- Salt to taste

Instructions:

1. Find a medium sized bowl enough to hold all the ingredients.

2. Add the creamy salad, cheese, and pimento cheese and mix.

3. Add salt and pepper to taste. Mix thoroughly for a few minutes.

Fried Tofu Chips

Tofus are some of the most nutritious sources of plant base protein. If you are a vegetarian on the Atkins diet, this is one of the most versatile sources of protein you can find. It can be taken with a lot of foods.

Ingredients:

- 16 ounces of tofu sliced to about ¼ of an inch
- Coconut or olive oil
- 1 tablespoon black pepper
- Salt to taste

Instructions:

1. Add about 1 to 1½ teaspoons of oil in a pan and heat.

2. Add the sliced tofus into the pan after the oil has heated for 30 seconds to a minute.

3. Do not let the tofus stick to each other, pile up and separate them and continue to turn them as they fry.

4. Fry the tofu until golden brown. Add some salt and pepper about a minute before you remove the pan from the stove.

5. You can serve with some melted cheese added on top of it.

Chapter 7: Staying Focused

The main goal for most people, who are on this meal plan, is to lose weight. Whatever your goal is, it is important to keep track of how well disciplined you've been. Here are a few tips:

- Write out a meal plan for at least two weeks or more and try and stick to it. You may check from time to time how disciplined you've been and adjust.

- Ensure you are getting enough carbohydrates and proteins, while at the same time, ensure you're not consuming them in excess. You may even weigh what you are eating to ensure you are getting the right amounts.

- If the main goal is to lose weight, you may check your weight after two weeks or so. The change in weight is very motivating. Avoid checking your weight daily. If you fail to see real change you may be de-motivated.

- If you're overweight, start with low impact cardio to avoid a burn out. You may then increase the intensity of the exercise progressively. This has proven to be a more effective strategy for most people.

Conclusion

Thank you again for purchasing this book!

Now I would like to ask for a *small* favor. I am self-published author, and if you liked my book, a review on Amazon would be a great help for me. This feedback will let me continue to write the kind of books that will help people and will let me improve.

Go to http://bit.ly/atkinscookreview to review, and thanks in advance for any kind of support!

Good luck!

– Sandra

Would You Like to Know More?

To check what are The 101 Tips That Burn Belly Fat Daily go to my page here:

=> http://projecteasylife.com/101tips <=

To see what are The 7 (Quick & Easy) Cooking Tricks To Banish Your Boring Diet go to my website here:

=> http://projecteasylife.com/7-tricks <=

[BONUS]

Preview of My Other Book, Wheat Belly Diet

(…)

Why Use the Wheat Belly Diet for the Best Results?

If you have tried and failed with other diets, perhaps you were not eliminating the right types of foods. Rethinking wheat has helped people to eliminate the harm it causes to your body. Getting rid of belly fat has thus far been a successful goal for people using the Wheat-Belly Diet.

Very few wheat-based foods are actually healthy for you to eat. The wheat used today, which Dr. Davis calls "Frankenwheat", is genetically modified, and it isn't the same wheat that your parents used to eat.

The modification of the wheat plant has allowed it to be thicker and shorter, so that it is more beneficial for farmers, and more resistant to disease. The bad aspect of this wheat is that it is not as nutritionally rich as conventional wheat, and can damage your health.

The glycemic index is higher in today's wheat than it is in sugar. Some candy bars have a healthier glycemic index than a slice of wheat bread. Glutens that are present in larger amounts in today's wheat cause cravings, and that leads to excess belly fat.

Dr. Davis says that you can expect better results from a wheat-free meal plan, because wheat is more than simply a gluten source. "Frankenwheat" affects the mind, by stimulating your appetite and it can cause depression and anxiety, especially for people who are overweight.

Giving up wheat will allow you to lose belly fat, and can also help in other health issues, such as those mentioned above. People are finally beginning to see the negative effects of today's wheat on their health, and those who stay with the Wheat Belly Diet often find benefits that they did not even expect.

(…)

To check out the rest of the book *Wheat Belly Diet*, go to Amazon here: http://bit.ly/wheatbellydiet

Check Out My Other Books

Below you'll find some of my other books that are popular on Amazon and Kindle as well. Simply go to the links below to check them out. Alternatively, you can visit my author page on Amazon to see other work done by me:

Author page: http://bit.ly/SandraWilliams

Gluten Free And Wheat Free Total Health Revolution

Wheat Belly Cookbook – *37 Wheat Free Recipes To Lose The Wheat And Have All-Day Energy* (http://bit.ly/bellycookbook)

Gluten Free – *The Gluten Free Diet For Beginners Guide, What Is Celiac Disease, How To Eat Healthier And Have More Energy* (http://bit.ly/glutenfreebook)

Gluten Free Cookbook – *30 Healthy And Easy Gluten Free Recipes For Beginners, Gluten Free Diet Plan For A Healthy Lifestyle* (http://bit.ly/gfreecookbook)

How To REALLY Set And Achieve Goals

Goals – *Setting And Achieving S.M.A.R.T. Goals, How To Stay Motivated And Get Everything You Want From Your Life Faster* (http://bit.ly/getsmartgoals)

Prevent And Reverse Diabetes Disease

Diabetes – *Diabetes Prevention And Symptoms Reversing* (http://bit.ly/diabetesguide)

Diabetic Cookbook – *30 Diabetes Diet Recipes For Diabetic Living, Control Low Sugar And Reverse Diabetes Naturally* (http://bit.ly/diabetic-cookbook)

Get Healthy, Have More Energy And Live Longer With Natural Paleo And Mediterranean Foods

Paleo – *The Paleo Diet For Beginners Guide, Easy And Practical Solution For Weight Loss And Healthy Eating* (http://bit.ly/healthypaleo)

Paleo Cookbook – *30 Healthy And Easy Paleo Diet Recipes For Beginners, Start Eating Healthy And Get More Energy With Practical Paleo Approach* (http://bit.ly/tastypaleo)

Mediterranean Diet – *Easy Guide To Healthy Life With Mediterranean Cuisine, Fast And Natural Weight Loss For Beginners* (http://bit.ly/mediterraneanbook)

Mediterranean Diet Cookbook – *30 Healthy And Easy Mediterranean Diet Recipes For Beginners* (http://bit.ly/mediterracookbook)

Extremely Fast Weight Loss With Low Carb Approach

Ketogenic Diet – *Easy Keto Diet Guide For Healthy Life And Fast Weight Loss, Heal Yourself And Get More Energy With Low Carb Diet* (http://bit.ly/ketodietbook)

Ketogenic Diet Cookbook – *30 Keto Diet Recipes For Beginners, Easy Low Carb Plan For A Healthy Lifestyle And Quick Weight Loss* (http://bit.ly/ketocookbook)

Amazing Weight Loss Tips, Tricks And Motivation

Weight Loss – *30 Tips On How To Lose Weight Fast Without Pills Or Surgery, Weight Loss Motivation And Fat Burning Strategies* (http://bit.ly/weightlosstipsbook)

Ultimate Guide To Diets – *Choose The Best Diet For Your Body, Live Healthy And Happy Life Without Supplements And Pills* (http://bit.ly/dietsbook)

The Obesity Cure – *How To Lose Weight Fast And Overcome Obesity Forever* (http://bit.ly/obesitybook)

Unique Beauty Tips Every Woman Should Know

Younger Next Month – *Anti-Aging Guide For Women* (http://bit.ly/beyoungerbook)

Hair Care And Hair Growth Solutions – *How To Regrow Your Hair Faster, Hair Loss Treatment And Hair Growth Remedies* (http://bit.ly/haircarebook)

Improve State Of Mind, Defeat Bad Feelings And Be Happy!

Anxiety Workbook – *Free Cure For Anxiety Disorder And Depression Symptoms, Panic Attacks And Social Anxiety Relief Without Medication And Pills* (http://bit.ly/anxietybook)

The Depression Cure – *Depression Self Help Workbook, Cure And Free Yourself From Depression Naturally And For Life* (http://bit.ly/depressioncurebook)

If the links do not work, for whatever reason, you can simply search for the titles on the Amazon website to find them. Best regards!

Made in the USA
San Bernardino, CA
05 October 2015